# MALGORZATA MAUCHI

# Not Another Diet Book: 10 Every Day Hacks to Help You Feel Fuller While Losing Weight and Staying Healthy for Life

# Contents

# 1

# Not Another Diet Book

10 Every Day Hacks to Help You Feel Fuller While Losing Weight and Staying Healthy for Life

Welcome!

I am excited that you have decided to dive in with me into this short, yet wholesome list of hacks that you can introduce in your daily life to improve your overall health while losing weight and feeling better about yourself; for life.

I have been working in the field of nutrition for over 12 years now and I have seen how our dietary and lifestyle choices can affect our overall health, our mood, our sleep and of course the obvious- our weight. In a nutshell, in order to live a healthier life and to avoid unwanted weight gain (or to achieve gradual and sustainable weight loss) you need to make adaptations in all aspects of your life. You've probably heard of superfoods that can do wonders for your health- like chia seeds, blueberries, turmeric, coffee, etc. And yes many of those so-called superfoods do have great health benefits, but they don't work in a vacuum- every information you read online or see on TV or any social media platform needs to be taken with a grain of salt and everything needs to be taken in moderation.

I am sure you've also seen a lot of advertisements for magic potions or pills that will do the trick of weight loss for you, and help shed unwanted inches fast. The truth is no diet pill or potion comes without a side effect and in all of those advertisements they say as a disclaimer that in order to achieve desirable results you must take it with a healthy diet and exercise. Well, why not just adjust the food and lifestyle choices without the unnecessary pills, potions or other magic tricks. Let's dive into those changes together. And yes there are so many fad diets to choose from, but which one is the right one? Which one really works and which one is just a quick fix with adverse long term effects? The word diet had a bad rep as well. Nobody really wants to be on a diet, but in reality we all are on some sort of diet that we decide to be on without knowing it is called a diet. Some people are on a See Food diet- I see food I eat food, that is a diet too. The one you want to be on is a wholesome, sustainable, not a fad short term diet but a lifelong committed healthy lifestyle one. The hacks listed in this book apply to all aspects of life but they are simple enough that anybody can do it.

# 2

# Hack # 1

**M**indful eating.

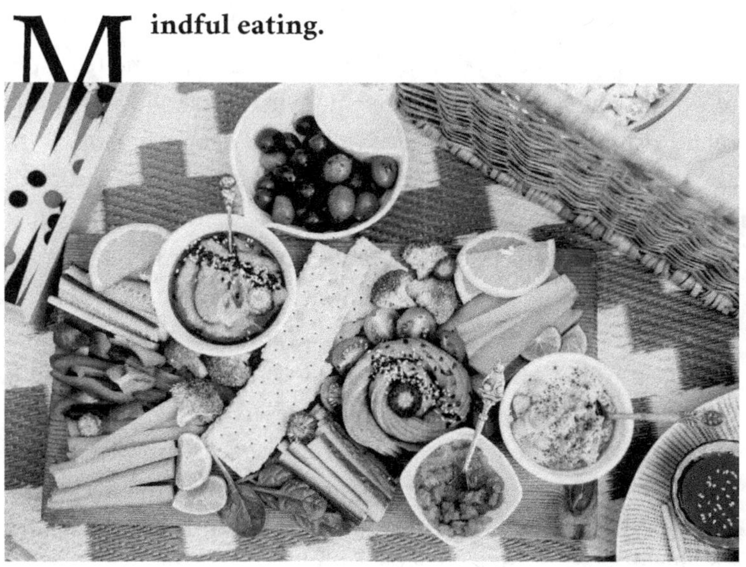

First let's look at our overall attitude towards ourselves and the food that we put into our bodies.  When you wake up in the morning and look in the mirror you see the person that is closest and dearest to you- literally. You should treat that person with love and respect, even when you are not satisfied with what's in front of you. Only when you begin to accept yourself and accept your body will you then start treating yourself like you deserve the best in life. Like the saying goes: healthy body- healthy mind. Which means that only when your mind is in the right place then your body will be in balance as well. The way you feel in your mind- whether you are happy, relaxed or stressed or depressed may show as physical signs on or inside your body.

Developing a healthy relationship with yourself is the first step to developing a healthy relationship with your food. A healthy relationship with food is multifaceted and deeply personal. It's about more than just the nutritional value of what we eat; it's about our attitudes and behaviors towards food and eating. Just like the relationship that you have with your inner self, your relationship to the food you eat should be positive, flexible, and nurturing, allowing for a balanced diet without imposing strict restrictions that can lead to guilt or stress. With that being said, what does it mean in practice? It involves listening to our body's hunger cues- which are key! How do we know when we are really hungry? If we are constantly bombarded with advertising of foods and snacks when we drive, at work on our computers, on our phones, through all social media platforms, and on TV it is hard to then distinguish which feelings of hunger come from the external vs internal cues. It is hard to shut all those external cues out and to listen to our inner voice that tells us what our body really needs, in terms of food, and when it really needs it. This is where mindful eating comes to place. It is important to learn to tune out the outside stimuli and focus on what our body really tells us. We want to eat for both nourishment and enjoyment, and not because we got lured in by an external cue.

Intuitively we all know which foods are good and which are not good for us and when we eat we know deep inside whether the food we are eating serves our bodies well and that it provides the nourishment that our bodies need or that it makes us feel good at the moment but long term it is not good for us. We know that when we eat vegetables, fruits and whole grains that it gives us vitamins, minerals and fiber that our bodies need. But we also know that when we drink soda, eat chips, cakes, and ice cream that it does not provide us with nutrients and that it can lead to weight gain and long term it can help develop diseases like diabetes, high blood pressure and heart disease.

In our approach to food we have to also recognize that our eating habits are influenced by a variety of factors like culture, tradition, and social interactions, and that these should be respected and integrated into our approach to food.

Ultimately, a healthy relationship with food is one that supports our overall well-being, both physically and mentally, and contributes to a fulfilling and enjoyable life. With all those factors in mind the food that you chose to eat should not give you a feeling of guilt, but a sense of joy and satisfaction.

# Hack # 2

**P**ortion Size is Key!

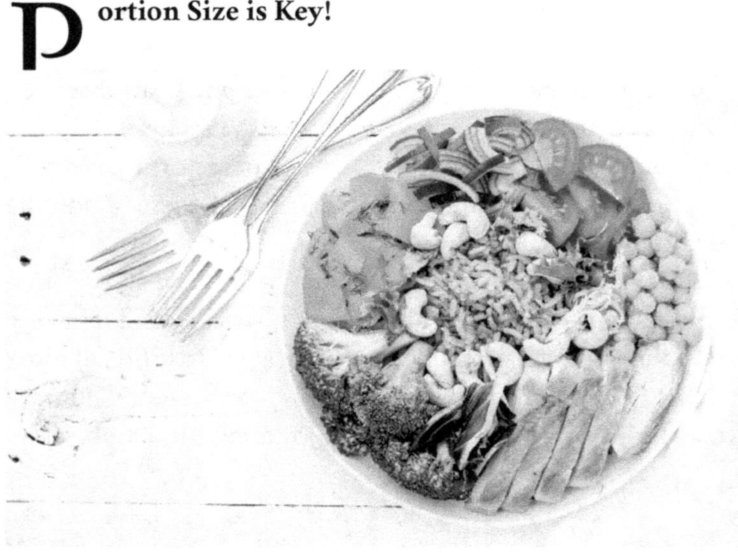

Understanding food portion sizes is crucial for maintaining a healthy diet and managing weight. A portion is the amount of food you choose to eat, which can vary greatly from person to person or meal to meal. In contrast, a serving size is a standardized unit of measuring food, such as those found on Nutrition Facts labels, and can help guide you on how much to eat. It's important to recognize that portion sizes can be larger than serving sizes, especially in restaurants, leading to overeating.

Over the years portion sizes of foods offered at restaurants, take outs and even packages of foods that we buy at grocery stores have increased slowly but significantly. An 8 oz glass bottle of soda used to be a standard size drink. Nowadays a 16 oz bottle is considered a standard size and many people chose to drink even larger portions like 20 or even a shocking 32 oz portion at a time. A regular size bagel found at a bakery nowadays is 2 times bigger than the one you could buy in the 1980s. If you order a take out dinner of steak, rice and a salad from a restaurant you will find that the portion of rice is 3 times bigger than what is recommended by USDA "My Plate" method. A portion of steak is also 2-3 times bigger than a recommended intake and the portion of salad is 3-4 times smaller than a recommended vegetable portion.

A "portion distortion"- the tendency to eat larger portions than recommended- is a recognized phenomenon where we no longer can rely on what we see and what we are offered as a standard of portions good for us and our health. We have to educate ourselves and be prepared to react accordingly to make better choices for our health. Being mindful of the portions we consume, measuring out servings at home, and being aware of the nutritional content can help in making healthier choices and avoiding portion distortion.

When preparing your meal at home make sure that you follow the My Plate guidelines: 3 oz of healthy protein (about a size of your hand without fingers), 1 cup of whole grain protein (about a size of a closed fist) and a rainbow of colors if it comes to vegetables; made the way you like it, that will cover half of your 9" standard plate. If you eat at a restaurant or order food out you can either eat some of the food and pack the rest for later or share it with a loved one or a friend It's a win-win situation where you save money on food while saving unnecessary calories.

# 4

# Hack # 3

**Choosing Lean Proteins like a PRO**

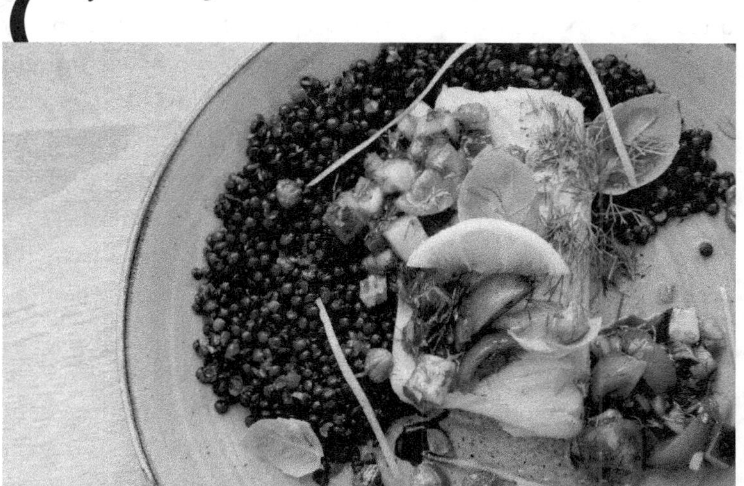

Protein is a crucial macronutrient that plays many roles in the body, such as building muscle, repairing tissue, and producing enzymes and hormones.  As important as protein is in our bodies there has been a recent boom in the western world for animal protein and the portions of animal proteins have gone way up making it seem, in some circles, as if it is the major source of food we should be consuming. As mentioned in the previous section a portion of starch should be an equivalent to the size of the palm of your hand.  A total daily average recommended intake of protein should be about 10-35% of your total food intake; based on how physically active you are. As you see it should be between 1/ 10 and 1/ 3 of what we eat, not more.

A variety of foods can provide healthy lean protein, including both animal and plant-based sources. Eggs are always getting mixed reviews due to their cholesterol content but after many studies they are still considered a wholesome/complete protein that offers a range of vitamins and minerals. Nuts like almonds and seeds are not only rich in protein but also provide healthy fats and fiber. Dairy products, particularly Greek yogurt, kefir and cottage cheese, are high in protein and calcium.  And my personal favorite plant-based options like lentils (which I personally love), beans, and quinoa are great for those following a vegetarian or vegan diet.

For those looking for lean meats, chicken breast or white fleshed fish like cod, haddock, bass or halibut, are excellent choices, packed with protein and essential nutrients. Red meat is high in protein but it also is rich in saturated fats which are not recommended for our heart health- for that reason consumption of red meat should be limited to 1-2 meals per week.

For those who are not vegans or vegetarians, including non-meat protein choices in their diets is also very important as those protein sources have a lower fat and cholesterol content, and a higher content of vitamins and minerals like iron, B vitamins and other micro nutrients. Incorporating a mix of protein sources into our daily diets and ensuring that a good percentage of our protein choices come from non-animal sources can detrimentally influence our optimal health and well being.

# 5

# Hack # 4

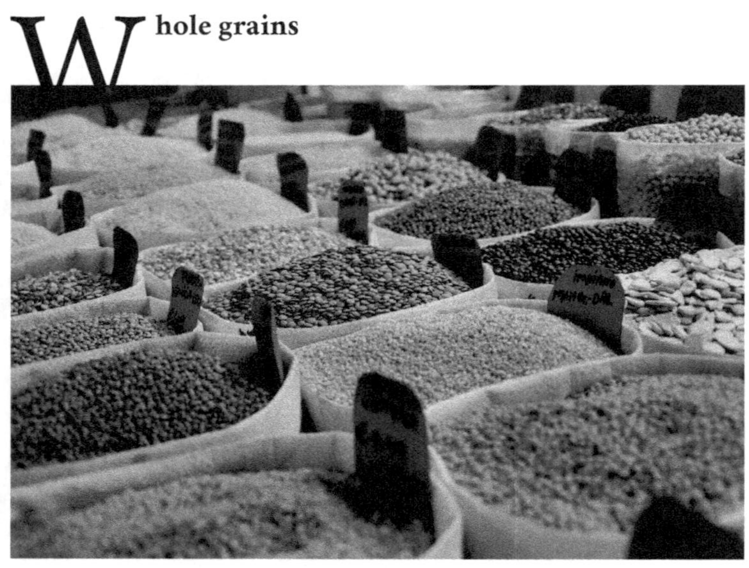

W hole grains

Choosing healthy carbohydrates is essential for a balanced diet. Carbohydrates are a primary source of energy, and selecting the right types can have a significant impact on your overall health. Whole, unprocessed or minimally processed carbs are the best choices. These include fruits, which provide natural sugars and fiber; whole grains like brown rice, oats, and quinoa, which offer complex carbs along with a range of nutrients; and vegetables, which are low in calories and high in vitamins and minerals. Legumes such as beans also offer a good mix of protein and complex carbohydrates.

All sources of carbohydrates are important in our diets but in this section we will focus on whole grains as part of a meal such as whole grain pasta, rice, quinoa, oats and whole grain breads. As mentioned in the previous chapter a healthy portion of carbohydrates is about the size of a fist or equals 1 cup. That is for a person who wants to maintain their weight. For somebody that is trying to lose weight a typical portion size of starch should be ½ cup of starch. It is not to say that if you eat less starch because you are trying to achieve weight loss you should eat less food overall. Foods like vegetables are not limited on any diet. Vegetables can be consumed in excess. It will be discussed in the next hack.

It is important to mention that there are starchy vegetables out there and that for the sake of weight loss or carbohydrate counting they are considered starch and not vegetables. Those vegetables are: potato, corn and legumes. Starchy vegetables need to be treated as a grain/starch and not a vegetable when preparing and plating your meal.

We all know that there are carbohydrates out there that are more appealing to us than others- for example french fries may seem more appealing than a baked potato but it is important to remember that in a frying process a lot of oil gets absorbed in the food and gets consumed. It's important to know that 1 tablespoon of oil has about 120 calories- an equivalent to the calories in 1 whole banana. For that reason cooking methods for our food also should be considered a factor in the overall health. Baking, boiling or broiling should be preferred methods.

It's important to opt for carbs that are high in fiber, as they can help regulate blood sugar levels and can contribute to a feeling of fullness, aiding in weight management. Additionally, choosing carbs that are rich in vitamins and minerals can support overall health. When planning meals, incorporating a variety of these healthy carbohydrate choices can ensure a well-rounded and nutritious diet.

# 6

# Hack # 5

**F**lood it all with veggies

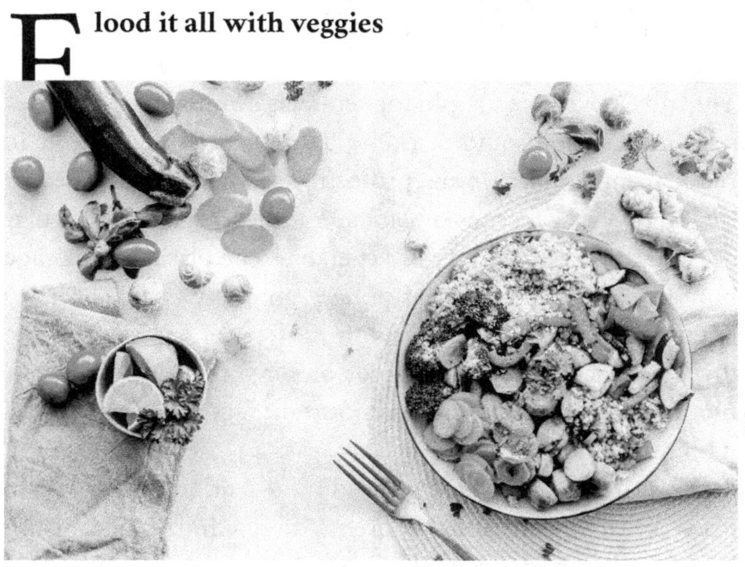

Vegetables are a cornerstone of a healthy diet, providing an array of nutrients essential for maintaining optimal health. They are rich in vitamins, minerals, and antioxidants, which are crucial for the body's various functions and disease prevention. For example, leafy greens like spinach and kale are high in vitamins A, C, and K, as well as minerals such as iron and calcium, which support vision, immune function, and bone health. Vegetables are also an excellent source of dietary fiber, which promotes digestive health and can aid in maintaining a healthy weight by providing a sense of fullness with fewer calories. They are low in calories, high in water content and high in fiber which can make you feel fuller for longer. That is why it is recommended to eat as many portions of vegetables per day as possible- the average intake recommendation is 3-5, but some studies suggest even 9 portions of vegetables to be consumed on a daily basis to achieve optimal health.

The diverse range of phytochemicals found in vegetables, such as flavonoids and carotenoids, play a significant role in reducing inflammation and protecting against chronic diseases, including certain types of cancer and heart disease. Regular consumption of a variety of vegetables can also help manage blood pressure due to their potassium content, which helps counteract the effects of sodium in the diet. Moreover, the low glycemic index of most vegetables makes them suitable for blood sugar management, an important factor for individuals with or at risk for diabetes.

Preparing vegetables can be done in numerous ways to preserve their nutritional content and maximize their health benefits. Steaming, roasting, and sautéing are methods that maintain the integrity of nutrients while also allowing for the addition of flavors that can make vegetables more appealing to a wide range of palates. It's also beneficial to consume vegetables that are in season, as they are often fresher and more nutrient-dense.

The importance of vegetables in our diet cannot be overstated. They provide essential nutrients that support overall health, protect against disease, and contribute to a balanced and nutritious diet. By making vegetables a regular part of our daily meals, we can enjoy a variety of health benefits that can enhance our quality of life and well-being.

# Hack # 6

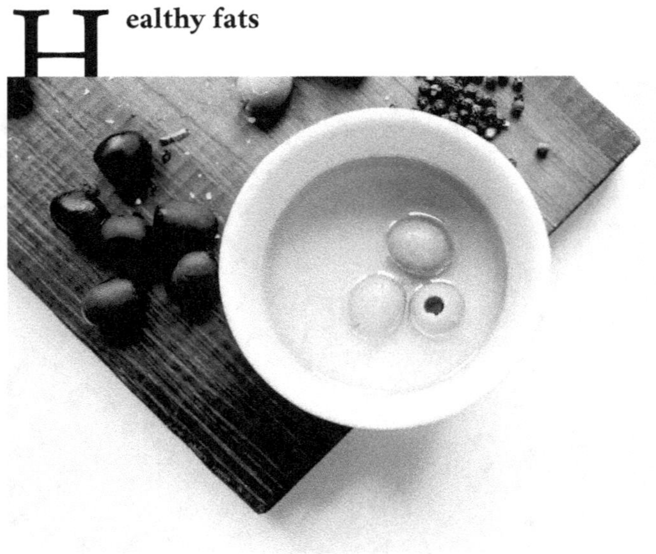

H ealthy fats

Healthy fats are essential for overall health, providing energy, supporting cell growth, and protecting organs. They also play a crucial role in helping the body absorb nutrients and produce important hormones. Some of the best sources of healthy fats include avocados, which are rich in monounsaturated fats and can help to increase good cholesterol levels while reducing bad cholesterol. Other sources include nuts, seeds, and olive oil, which contain a mix of monounsaturated and polyunsaturated fats that contribute to heart health. Fatty fish, such as salmon and mackerel, are high in omega-3 fatty acids, known for their anti-inflammatory properties and benefits to cardiovascular health. It's important to incorporate a variety of these fats into a balanced diet to reap the full range of health benefits they offer.

On the other hand it is important to try and stay away from the fats that may be detrimental to our health. Animal fat has been shown to have a negative impact on our health in the form of heart disease. We should refrain from eating deep fried foods and opt for healthier cooking methods like baking, boiling, broiling and lately very popular- air frying.

When adding oil to cooking the best choices are olive oil, avocado oil or grape seed oil as they have been shown to have the best health benefits and also the latter 2 of the 3 have a relatively high smoke point and will not burn the food.

# 8

# Hack # 7

Healthy Snacks, even on the go…

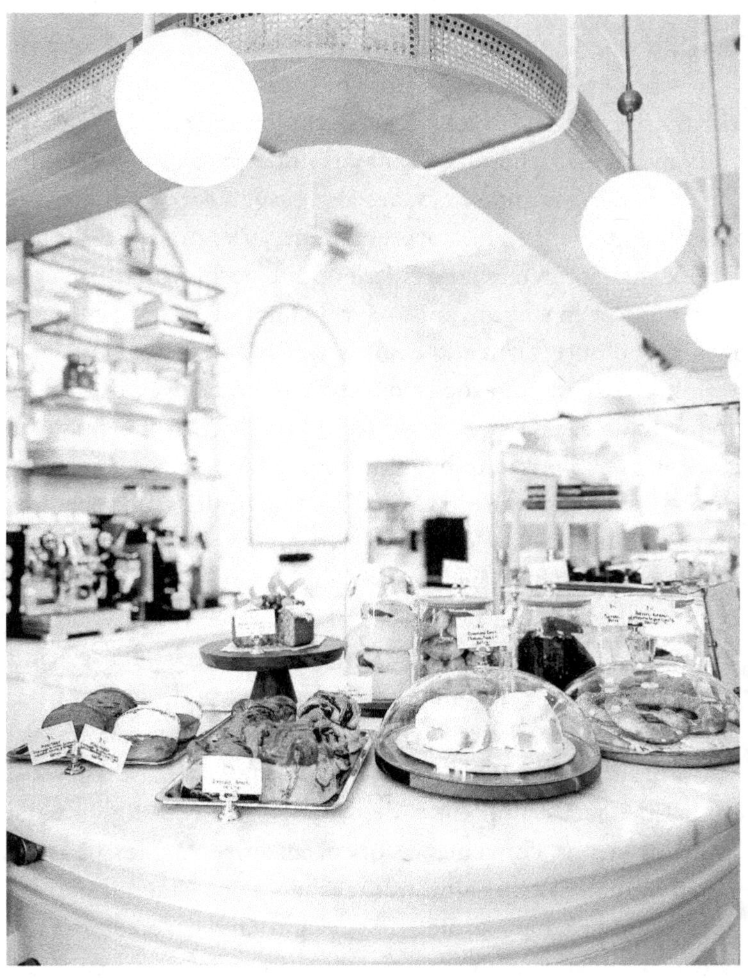

For those leading a busy lifestyle, finding snacks that are both healthy and convenient can be a challenge. However, there are numerous options that can fit into a hectic schedule. Packable snacks like Oatmeal bars, Chocolate-Caramel Energy Bars and Air-Fryer Crispy Chickpeas offer a balance of taste and nutrition, perfect for those living on-the-go. Roasted chickpeas, in particular, are a great source of protein and fiber, making them an excellent snack to keep you energized throughout the day. Fresh fruits like bananas and apples, or vegetables like baby carrots and celery, are also easy to carry and provide essential nutrients. For a protein boost, jerky or single-serving Greek yogurt can be a convenient option, just be sure to choose varieties low in sodium and sugar. Combining these with nuts or almond butter can add healthy fats and additional protein, keeping you full and focused. Remember, the key to healthy snacking is to choose foods that are as close to their natural state as possible, and to be mindful of portion sizes.

In my daily commute to work I find that healthy snack choices can be found in the least expected places. I've heard those voices in the past - where I live there are no good food/snack options. I found out to be not entirely true. When you walk into a convenience store or a gas station in search of snacks it is important what your mind is already set on getting. If you are looking for high fat, high calorie snacks or high sugary snacks you will surely find them. But here is a list of snacks that I most often find that are nutritious, delicious and on a healthy side and available in most convenience, or corner stores: apples, bananas, roasted nut mixes or almonds, cashews or pistachios, string cheese, oatmeal bars, protein bars, yogurt and baked chips. You will also find a whole range of unhealthy snacks but again it is important what your mind is already set on getting. Not only you will find a whole gamut of unhealthy snack options but also a whole fridge full of sugary drink options. If you are easily persuaded or you are extremely hungry you may fall victim to one of those snacks that you know will not serve you well. Try to always choose what is best for your body. In terms of drinks-water, seltzer water or flavored seltzer are your best choices-there is so much unnecessary added sugar in sweetened drinks, it is truly not worth dealing with the consequences of the added sugar consumed in drinks. Diet soda has been linked to an increase in appetite so it is also not recommended if the effect is- you being more hungry after drinking it.

It is not to say that you can never treat yourself to snacks that you like the taste of but know that are not good for you but it should be an exception to your rule, a treat and not a daily occurrence.

# 9

# Hack # 8

Move it daily

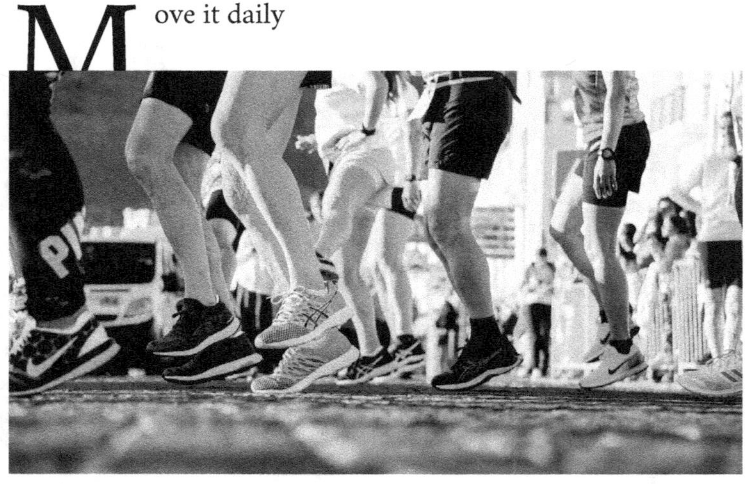

Daily physical activity is essential for maintaining good health and well-being.  As highlighted by health experts, engaging in regular exercise can have profound effects on mental and physical health. According to The Physical Activity Guidelines for Americans we should all get involved in 150 minutes minimum of physical activity on a weekly basis. That's 20 minutes 7 days a week or 30 min 5 days a week - minimum. Out of that 2 days out of a week we should do muscle strengthening activities. This is a bare minimum amount of physical activity that we should be doing. Studies suggest that many people need more physical activity than 30 min per day to maintain a healthy weight over time. Some studies suggest 45-60 min of physical activity is needed to achieve optimal health and to keep a healthy weight in check. The type of physical activity you engage in does not have to be structured if it does not fit your lifestyle. For example: 10 minutes of stretching is an equivalent of walking a football field, 20 minutes of vacuuming is like walking a mile, 30 minutes of grocery shopping is already 30 minutes of walking done. If you have stairs at home you can run up and down for 10 minutes. All the little movements throughout the day count.

As per The Physical Activity Guidelines for Americans just from a single session of physical activity we get the benefits of blood pressure reduction, improved insulin sensitivity, improved sleep, reduced anxiety symptoms, and some cognitive function improvement on the day that it is performed, it also releases endorphins thus making us feel good.

Physical activity can help prevent a range of diseases and enhance the overall quality of life. Physical activity boosts mood, combats disease, and promotes better sleep, among other benefits. For instance, it can increase high-density lipoprotein (HDL) cholesterol, the "good" cholesterol, and decrease unhealthy triglycerides, which in turn can lower the risk of cardiovascular diseases. Moreover, it's a key factor in weight management and can improve bone and muscle strength, making daily tasks easier and reducing the risk of falls in older adults. The World Health Organization also emphasizes the role of physical activity in preventing noncommunicable diseases and improving mental health, quality of life, and well-being. Therefore, incorporating physical activity into daily routines is a vital step towards a healthier life.

# 10

# Hack # 9

**G**et plenty of sleep

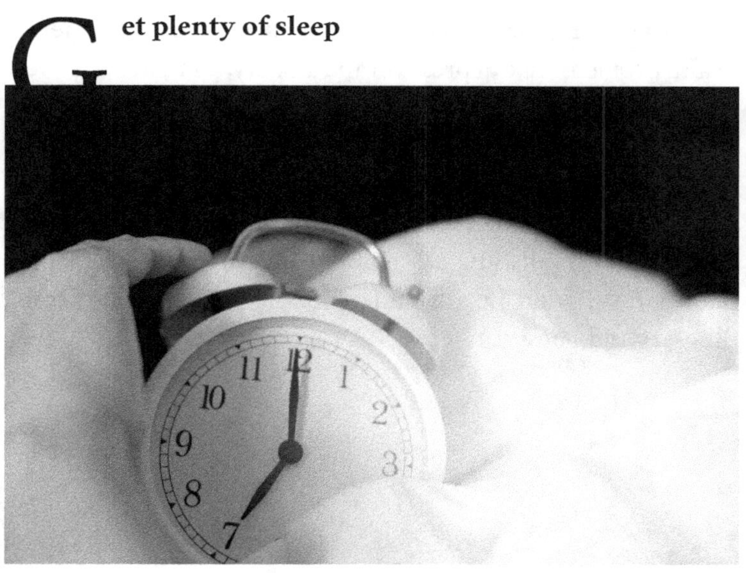

Sleep patterns have a profound impact on overall health, influencing various aspects of physical and mental well-being.

Consistent, quality sleep contributes to cognitive functions such as memory, attention, and decision-making. How much sleep is enough sleep? For all adults a good night's sleep is 7-8 hours, for teenagers is 8-10 hours. Conversely, irregular or insufficient sleep can lead to a range of health issues, including cardiovascular disease, obesity, and diabetes. For instance, sleep deprivation can increase stress hormones, which in turn may raise resting heart rate and blood pressure, potentially leading to long-term heart health issues. That same stress hormone - cortisol has been linked to weight gain, that is why it is so very important to get a good night sleep to prevent weight gain and the diseases associated with it like diabetes, heart disease, high blood pressure among all others.

Furthermore, sleep deficiency has been linked to mental health problems like depression and anxiety, and can even affect emotional regulation and behavior.

It's not just the quantity of sleep that matters, but also the quality; uninterrupted sleep allows the brain to process and consolidate memories, and the body to repair and rejuvenate. Therefore, establishing a regular sleep pattern is crucial for maintaining good health and reducing the risk of chronic illnesses and obesity.

# 11

# Hack # 10

**R**eading Labels vs Label Free foods

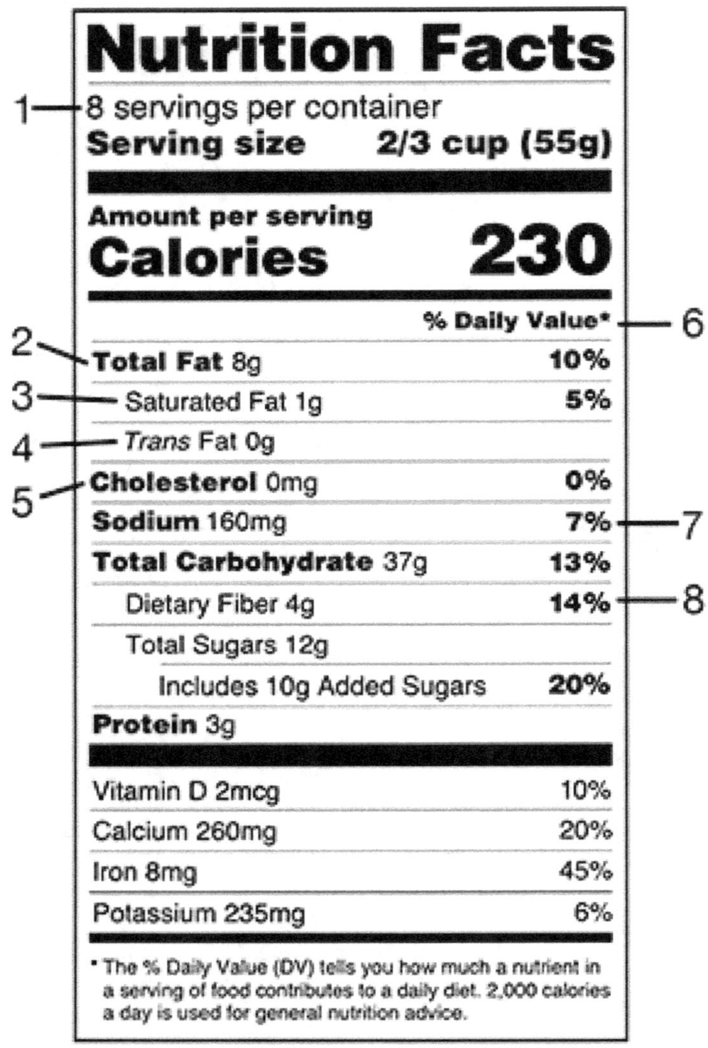


Reading food labels is an essential skill for making informed dietary choices. The Nutrition Facts label on packaged foods provides vital information about the nutritional content of the food inside. To effectively read a food label, start by checking the serving size and the number of servings per container, as all the nutritional information is based on one serving. Pay attention to the calories per serving, which indicates how much energy you'll get from consuming one serving of the food. Look at the nutrients, focusing on those you may want to get more of, like dietary fiber, vitamin D, calcium, iron, and potassium.

Conversely, you may want to limit the foods with nutrients like saturated fat, trans fat, sodium, and added sugars. The Percent Daily Value (%DV) helps you understand how much a nutrient in a serving of food contributes to a daily diet, based on a 2,000 calorie per day diet- which is a standard for all adults, but in reality not all adults need 2000 calories per day, based on their height and physical activity level.

A %DV of 5% or less is low for all nutrients, those you want to limit and those you want to consume in greater amounts. A %DV of 20% or more is high. This information can help you discern if a food aligns with your nutritional needs or dietary restrictions.

You may have heard the term "shopping the perimeter" of the store. It means that when you enter the store you will find fruits and vegetables first- this is where most of your shopping should be done. Then you move to the back of the store where you find all your proteins and then you head to the other end of the store where you find all your dairy and eggs. Anything in the center aisles is considered less necessary, most likely have a higher content of added ingredients,added sugars, added salt, and may be less nutritious. The foods around the perimeter that have no nutrition fact labels are highly desirable as they are more natural, have less additives and are overall better for our health. If you are shopping for foods with labels look at the ingredient list- anything with 5 ingredients or less is a good choice overall. Stay away from food coloring and foods with chemicals that you don't know or can't pronounce.

Foods which by law do not require nutrition fact labels are often considered healthier because they typically include whole, unprocessed foods like fresh fruits and vegetables. These foods are rich in essential nutrients, including vitamins, minerals, and fiber, without the added sugars, fats, and preservatives commonly found in processed foods. The absence of a label signifies that the food is in its natural state, providing the body with the purest form of nutrition. While nutrition labels can help consumers make informed choices about packaged foods, focusing on foods without labels can lead to a more natural, whole-foods-based diet, which many health experts recommend for optimal health.

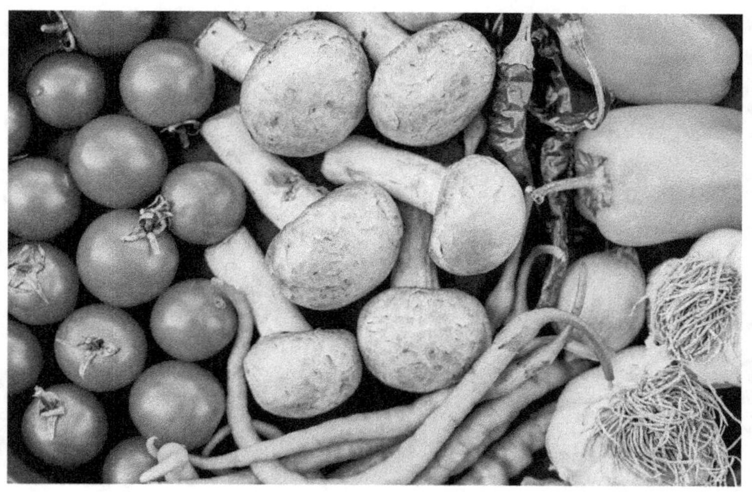

# 12

# Conclusion

As we reach the end of our journey where we find out what daily hacks we can do to optimize our health for life, it becomes clear that true wellness is not just a destination, but a lifelong commitment. This book is a brief illustration of a more complex concept of a mindful approach to life and food, not a diet, of prioritizing wholesome foods on a daily basis, of incorporating daily physical activity, and getting sufficient and restful sleep to achieve lifelong health and desirable weight.

The bottom line of this book is that there is no one simple easy solution to achieve lifelong health and wellness. There is no one aspect of life that can be quickly fixed, a pill added and there we have it, all done. It is a multifaceted process where no stone of life can be unturned. At the same time none of it is a hard chore and no food should feel like it's an obligation for us to eat it. We can all make it fun and it can be smoothly incorporated into our daily routines no matter what our cultural background, gender or age. We can all benefit from the same 10 hacks of being mindful about our food, eating with portion control in mind, choosing lean proteins, whole grains, bountiful and colorful veggies, healthy snacks, and finishing it off with sufficient physical activity that make us feel better and happier and finally get a good night sleep to gain the energy to do it all again tomorrow.

If you found this book helpful I would appreciate it if you could please leave a favorable review on Amazon. Thank you.

# 13

# Resources:

Food and mood – *Healthy Minds*. (n.d.). Healthy Minds. https://www.healthyminds.services/support/articles /food-and-mood

Brooks, J. W. (2023, May 19). *Mindful Eating: 3 steps to feast with your senses and eat more healthfully*. Gaples Institute. https://www.gaplesinstitute.org/mindful-eating-3-steps-to-fe ast-with-your-senses-and-eat-more-healthfully/?gad_source= 1&gclid=CjwKCAjwr7ayBhAPEiwA6EIGxLZm5sP3NxXBH_ tnRxZCIYzUpKFpjMIVs_rot7pUZ_vH7s-deqrQ9RoCkw4Q AvD_BwE

*Portion size versus serving size.* (2023, December 18). www.heart.org. https://www.heart.org/en/healthy-living /healthy-eating/eat-smart/nutrition-basics/portion-size-vers us-serving-size

Ld, L. W. M. R. (2022, January 18). *Understanding 'Portion distortion' and learning how to eat mindful servings.* Healthline. https://www.healthline.com/nutrition/portion-distortion#:~:

text=Portions%20have%20grown%20in%20astounding,is%20
not%20unique%20to%20bagels.

*USDA MyPlate What is MyPlate?* (n.d.). https://www.myplate.g
ov/eat-healthy/what-is-myplate

DiGiacinto, J. (2023, November 6). *Top 13 lean protein foods.*
Healthline. https://www.healthline.com/nutrition/lean-protei
n-foods

Phillips, J. A. (2021). Dietary Guidelines for Americans,
2020–2025. *Workplace Health & Safety, 69*(8), 395. https://doi.
org/10.1177/21650799211026980
Piercy, K. L., Troiano, R. P., Ballard, R. M., Carlson, S. A.,
Fulton, J. E., Galuska, D. A., George, S. M., & Olson, R. D. (2018).
The physical activity guidelines for Americans. *JAMA, 320*(19),
2020. https://doi.org/10.1001/jama.2018.14854

Activity, M. P. (2020, November 25). *WHO guidelines on physical
activity and sedentary behaviour.* https://www.who.int/publicat
ions/i/item/9789240015128

*How sleep affects your health | NHLBI, NIH.* (2022, June 15).
NHLBI, NIH. https://www.nhlbi.nih.gov/health/sleep-dep
rivation/health-effects

*How much sleep is enough | NHLBI, NIH.* (2022, March 24).
NHLBI, NIH. https://www.nhlbi.nih.gov/health/sleep-dep
rivation/how-much-sleep

*Reading food labels.* (n.d.). Saint Luke's Health System. https://w

ww.saintlukeskc.org/health-library/reading-food-labels

ABC News. (2009, February 9). *What does "Shop the Perimeter" mean?* https://abcnews.go.com/Health/WellnessResource/story?id=6762968

www.ingramcontent.com/pod-product-compliance
Lightning Source LLC
Chambersburg PA
CBHW071553260726
48653CB00007BA/3056